Yoga

A Yogi's Explanation and Instructions

Chandra Dhopatkar

Indirect Knowledge Limited

Jackson, Michigan

Indirect Knowledge Publishing
4023 Briggs Ct.
Jackson, MI/49201
www.indirectknowledge.com

Yoga/ Chandra Dhopatkar. -- 1st ed.
ISBN 9798708691729

Dedicated to my wife Jennifer Bonilla

"Words are the most powerful drug used by mankind."

— Rudyard Kipling

CONTENTS

CHAPTER 1

What Is Yoga?

Yoga is an evolving science concerned with the study of wholesome human well-being. The word "yoga" comes from the Sanskrit root - "yuj" meaning unity. Yoga is a set of interrelated physical, emotional, and psychological practices or disciplines that originated in ancient India. Yoga can be added to a daily routine to increase flexibility, health, and strength.

There are different schools of yoga. (The term "yoga" refers to the physical postures.) In the United States, the most popular form of yoga is Vinyasa yoga, which is sometimes called "flow yoga." Vinyasa yoga combines many physical and breathing exercises with dynamic stretching movements. Vinyasa yoga consists of a series of gentle, flowing stretches, which can be repeated in as many sessions as necessary for the participant's physical condition and flexibility.

Vinyasa yoga combines a meditative focus with energetic activities that connect the body, mind, and spirit. Many proponents of yoga see it as a way to realize the mind-body relationship through a series of physical poses that stretch, stabilize, and improve the body. The eight limbs of yoga include various poses (called chakras) that stretch and strengthen all the internal organs and tissues of the body.

Vinyasa yoga practitioners view these internal organs and tissues as mirrors of our true nature - seeing, feeling, breathing, and being in alignment with our true Self, the supreme creator.

Many yoga sutras emphasize the significance of each chakra, or limb, in relation to the others. Chakra theory is the basis of many of the deeper aspects of yoga. For example, the first chakra is associated with Dharana or the third eye, located in the top center of the forehead. Hara yoga means wisdom; therefore, knowing the placement of the various chakras helps a student to develop a clear understanding of his or her own mind and self. The second chakra, known as the Brahma chakra, is related to physical and mental control.

Meditation is another important aspect of yoga that relates to the physical postures. Most yoga teachers begin their classes with meditation and contemplation exercises. These techniques help the participants to calm their minds and bodies, allowing them to focus on the breathing techniques during the meditation classes. The goal of meditation is to allow the mind and body to achieve unity and harmony through inner stillness. Meditation also allows the mediators to free themselves from physical and psychological stress by allowing the mind to release its concerns to the highest power within.

A well-balanced diet that includes a variety of whole foods is recommended for individuals who are practicing yoga on a regular basis. Most yoga practitioners (called yogis) are vegetarian, consuming only milk and dairy along with vegetables and grains. Because yoga positions can be quite strenuous, a healthy diet is essential to achieving the desired results. Common vegetables and fruits, coupled with whole grains and plant protein sources such as legumes and lentils help to improve overall well-being and provide much needed energy for a person doing yoga exercises.

Yoga can benefit most people physically and emotionally. The various yoga postures are said to help with improving strength, flexibility and stamina. Many yoga experts note that yoga is especially beneficial for people who participate in physically demanding sports or those who are recovering from an illness or injury. The yoga positions help to enhance balance and improve overall strength. It is also noted that yoga postures can help relieve stress and increase awareness. This can be especially beneficial for individuals who are working toward quitting smoking, alcohol or drugs, or who are trying to establish a healthy relationship with their fellow coworkers or neighbors.

It should be noted that all yoga postures, whether they are practiced individually or in combination with other forms of meditation, are designed to improve both the body and mind. However, it is important to remember that each of these elements has its own purpose and how it affects each other. A good example would be that while meditation helps to develop concentration, postures help to improve flexibility.

CHAPTER 2

Yoga For Those With Medical Conditions

Yoga is a unique collection of mental, emotional, and physical practices or philosophies that originated in ancient India. It uses breathing exercises to focus the mind. This practice is also used as a form of exercise to increase strength, flexibility, balance, and stamina. Yoga consists of numerous branches such as Raja Yoga, Hatha Yoga, Jnana Yoga, Kundalini Yoga, Tantra Yoga, Ashtanga Yoga, etc. Yoga combines physical exercises with meditative techniques to attain a sense of spirituality.

There are various aspects of yoga postures that should be considered before enrolling for any class or course. For instance, all students should seek out yoga instructors who have experience teaching correct posture and proper form. As such, yoga instructors should be able to ensure that students maintain a correct posture through explanation and demonstration. All yoga postures should be performed correctly so that the body maintains proper alignment while performing the exercise. Proper posture and alignment help to reduce back pain and sciatica and to increase one's overall sense of health.

Students should also seek out a yoga instructor who is experienced in teaching yoga postures to those suffering from medical conditions such as diabetes, heart disease, asthma, COPD, epilepsy, blood pressure, etc. These medical conditions require different postures and modifications of the practice that should only be conducted by an instructor certified in these matters. In addition, yoga instructors should also offer instruction regarding relaxation techniques such as meditation and deep breathing. Meditation is essential to achieving peace of mind while meditating as it helps to calm the mind.

The poses in yoga should not be used for weight loss purposes, as they are too strenuous. They should only be used for specific medical conditions and for the proper form of each pose. Excessive stretching of the muscles can lead to injury as well as to poor posture. If you have any medical conditions, or if you have decided to learn yoga postures because of those conditions, then you must make sure you are learning them from a qualified instructor.

Ashtanga yoga is a style of continuous flow yoga that originated in India and is often called Hatha yoga or "eight limbs movements." Hatha yoga combines yoga movements with simple asanas, breathing exercises, and meditation to bring about physical and mental balance. It aims to develop a state of awareness and tranquility by focusing on the body's subtle movements, breathing patterns, sensations, and thought processes. The asana, or postures, are regulated by a central mantra or word that is spoken in order to obtain a proper form and regulate the body's energy flow.

Some people who have decided to practice yoga postures due to medical conditions are surprised to find they improve their health and energy levels even though they are not experiencing any pain. Medical studies have shown that yoga can improve the immune system and ward off certain illnesses, such as cancer. When the immune system is functioning properly, the individual is also less susceptible to colds and other viral illnesses. These studies have shown that yoga instructors can teach seniors how to use certain postures that can actually strengthen the immune system. In addition, yoga can improve overall flexibility and strengthen muscles and bones.

CHAPTER 3

Yoga As a Form of Meditation

Yoga is a group of spiritual, psychological, and physical practices or disciplines that originated in ancient India. The word "yoga" actually means "to join," and is usually used to refer to physical yoga. Today yoga has grown to become a very popular exercise regimen. Yoga is one of the many six pastry schools of Hindu philosophical traditions.

Yoga is commonly practiced in conjunction with meditation techniques. This type of combination is referred to as "the yoga combination." There are several different levels of practice, from beginners to advanced practitioners, and this varies widely according to tradition. The ultimate goal of yoga is to merge mind, body, and spirit into a unified whole.

Meditation is the foundation of yoga, but yoga itself does not focus on meditation specifically. In fact, many instructors suggest that meditation is done before yoga exercises in order to achieve the maximum benefit from the meditative practices. The primary focus of meditation is breathing and in particular the breathing techniques known as pranayama. These breathing techniques are designed to reduce stress and promote relaxation.

Another technique common in both yoga and meditation is movement. Yoga can be practiced individually, but it is much more effective when performed in group settings. Hatha and Jnana yoga postures are good examples of yoga movements that are commonly practiced yoga in conjunction with meditation techniques. Some of these postures, such as the half moon and upward facing dog, require more focus than do others, such as the seated shoulder stand, but all postures promote a sense of well-being.

Most people who first begin practicing yoga don't realize how much connection there actually is between yoga and meditation. Once the connection is made, however, it becomes easier to integrate yoga and meditation into each day's activities. For instance, when you engage in yoga while taking deep breaths, you are really breathing in through your nose and out through your mouth. This combination allows you to deepen your concentration and bring about a sense of calmness and relaxation.

Another important factor to consider when learning to meditate is proper form. Proper form is crucial for consistent effectiveness, and it is important for the form of your breathing as well. Breathing in and out slowly and deeply through your nose while looking straight ahead (with your back straight) while your shoulders follow suit will help you achieve proper form. Your physical awareness as you practice proper form during yoga postures will help your mind stay focused as well. If you find yourself drifting here and there during a yoga session, it may be a good idea to remind yourself to observe proper form, or have someone with you during the exercises to assist you in holding your breathing in while your mind wanders.

One of the key elements of both yoga postures and correct breathing technique is reducing stress. In fact, yoga instructors recommend that their students practice meditation and breathing techniques daily in order to lower stress levels. If you want to reduce stress levels, you need to practice yoga postures on a regular basis, even if you don't feel stressed out. Regularly practicing yoga will allow your muscles to tighten up and become more stabilized, and the deep breathing exercises practiced while doing your yoga postures will help you relax more effectively.

Overall, if you practice consistently enough, yoga can lead to a more relaxed body and mind. When you combine proper breathing techniques with postures that are meant to reduce stress, you will experience a new level of inner peace. The more you meditate and breathe, the more relaxed you will become, which will allow you to live a better quality of life. You can also learn more about meditation and the art of yoga from a yoga instructor, or talk with others who practice the art of yoga on a daily basis.

CHAPTER 4

Yoga for Beginners: A Complete Pathway

Yoga is an ancient set of spiritual, mental, and physical practices or philosophies that originate in ancient India. The word "yoga" comes from the Sanskrit origin, meaning "to join." Yoga is now one of the many six worldwide strands of Indian intellectual traditions. It is said to bring together all of our senses, allowing us to perceive life in a whole new way.

Yoga is considered one of the healing sciences because it has been proven to relieve tension and stress. It improves overall health, helps us become calmer, strengthens our mental faculties, develops self-control, and balances our energy systems. Most importantly, yoga can help us develop self-awareness and improve our self-image. It is important for those with stress-filled careers to incorporate yoga into their daily routine, as well as those with a hectic lifestyle. Yoga is not just a physical exercise; rather, it is an ideal way to enhance our mental well-being.

Yoga has also been shown to be effective in the treatment of some illnesses, such as chronic pain and depression. In fact, yoga may prove to be a useful adjunct to standard medicine in the treatment of these and other ailments. The power yoga poses (Poses) have been known to increase circulation, relax muscles, regulate respiration, strengthen the tendons and ligaments of the body, increase stamina, increase strength, improve concentration, improve mood, improve sleep quality, build strength and flexibility, and open the energy channels. Yoga can be practiced by people of all ages, including pregnant women, children, the elderly, athletes, and those with illnesses or physical disabilities. Some of the more popular yoga poses include sun salutation (Surya-Vilasana), which stretch the back and chest; child (Shiro-Tribe), which are good for blood flow; forward bend (Bikram Yoga), which stretches the legs; plank (Iyengar), which lengthen the spine; half moon (Svadhyaya), which strengthens the abdominal muscles; twisting (Ustrasana), which stretches the muscles of the trunk; shoulder stand (Makarasana), which tones and tightens the shoulders; and modifications of the above poses.

Many of yoga's poses are performed with a comfy chair or on the floor. A beginner yoga class begins with gentle stretches and slow, rhythmic breathing exercises. The yoga class then moves toward a position of meditation, through which regulated breathing exercises are taught. These breathing exercises help the mind to settle into the body and allow students to connect their body and breath.

The sequence of postures is then paired with meditation. The goal of practicing yoga is to achieve inner enlightenment, called dharana. The postures are then followed by controlled breathing exercises, which gradually deepen and expand the body's consciousness. The postures of power yoga include sun salutation (Surya-Vilasana), which is soothing and calming; forward bend (Paschimottanasana), which lengthens the spine; and back bend (Cresting Sun Pose), which is very useful for relieving stress and tension in the body. Power yoga practitioners often combine these postures with other breathing exercises such as Kapalabhati.

Another way to view yoga is to consider it as an art form, or a journey along the complete path. The word yoga means "to unite" and "to work," and this union of mind and body comes together in a meaningful way. As this total path is studied and practiced, the individual leaves the self and creates a new, deeper self with each new step along the way.

If you are interested in learning power yoga poses, it's important to remember that beginners should begin with gentle poses, which are easier to learn. Power yoga poses are challenging, though. Beginners should practice these poses slowly and cautiously, using the props provided. Don't do any pose more than you can handle comfortably, particularly if you experience pain. You can stretch and experiment with various poses at your own pace.

If you want to get more from your hatha yoga routine, you can add various other aspects of yoga to your workout. For instance, you can focus on the breath, which many people overlook while practicing yoga. You can also try adding meditation or relaxation techniques. Some people enjoy the sound of flowing water during their workout, which can be achieved by practicing seated and standing poses (water yoga). And don't forget to have fun!

CHAPTER 5

Becoming a Yoga Instructor

Yoga has many definitions; however, the definition given below pertains to the physical aspect of it. Yoga is an array of mental, emotional, and spiritual practices or beliefs that originate from the ancient Indian discipline of the yogis. It is one the six mainstic schools of Indian yogic philosophies. The term itself derives from the Sanskrit word "yuj", which means union. Yoga combines breathing exercises, meditation, physical movements, and the study of yoga philosophy and ethics.

Many people are intrigued by this all-encompassing subject. For one who does not know much about yoga, it would be difficult to understand the essence of all the disciplines within it. There are those who believe that yoga is strictly a physical exercise routine, while others who adhere to the philosophy believe that it is more than that. Still, there are numerous yoga classes that will cater to all levels of experience.

Yoga originated from the Sanskrit term "yuj" meaning joining. The word is thought to be derived from the Hindu phrase, "to join with". In other words, yoga is believed to be a path of union between the spirit and the body. Because of its spirituality, it has been practiced for thousands of years.

A yoga instructor must be a qualified practitioner who has studied yoga for a minimum of three years. They must also receive formal training from an organization recognized by the American Board of Yoga, or the International Federation of Teachers of Yoga. Many organizations offer certification programs to teach yoga. If you choose to become a yoga instructor, you will complete a teacher training program. Some colleges and universities offer a yoga teacher training program that can be completed in as little as five months.

Upon completing your yoga teacher training, you will have the necessary knowledge and skills to start instructing yoga sessions. Most colleges and universities will require you to demonstrate your yoga skills before being officially licensed to teach yoga. Your academic background and practice on the yoga mats before taking your yoga teacher certification exam are very important factors when preparing for your test.

Once you have passed your test and received your official certification as a yoga teacher, you will need to find a teacher job. You may feel pressure from your peers at school or from the administration office if you are still having trouble finding a job. Keep in mind that there are a variety of different types of positions available in the field of yoga. It is important to be aware of your options and choose the one that fits best with your life and skill set. A career as a yoga teacher is very stable and pays well compared to other professions.

The job market for yoga instructors is vast and diverse. If you are interested in becoming a yoga instructor, it is important to do some initial research. There are many online resources available for yoga instructor training. Many schools are happy to provide online resources and classes. If you live in a small town or community, chances are there are not enough schools to meet your needs.

The Internet can also be a valuable resource when it comes to finding yoga instructor training. There are numerous online yoga classes available. Many of them are designed to be very interactive, which can make learning yoga more enjoyable. If you are thinking about teaching yoga to students in another country, you may want to take a virtual yoga class to see how you would do in real life. The instructor responsibilities will be very different than what you would experience in a traditional class.

ABOUT THE AUTHOR

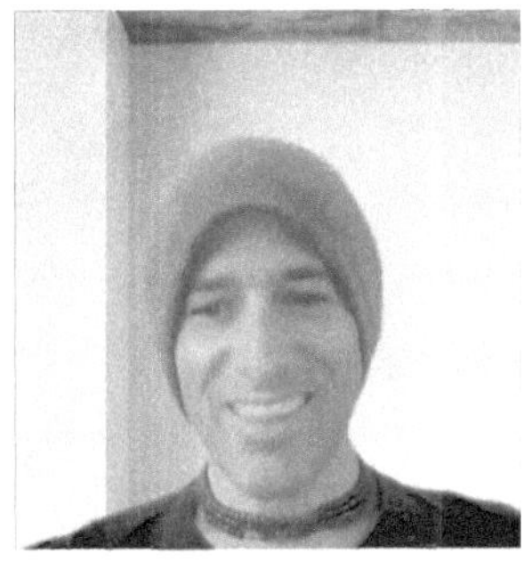

Chandra Dhopatkar is a content writer who formerly worked as an internet marketer. A content writer by day and a home chef by night, he is loath to discuss himself in the third person but can be persuaded to do so from time to time.

Learn more about him:

www.indirectknowledge.com